DASH DIET COOKBOOK

LOW-SODIUM RECIPES TO REDUCE YOUR WEIGHT AND LOWER YOUR BLOOD PRESSURE

JENNA JENKINS

Table of Contents

Turkey and Cumin Broccoli

Preparation time: 10 minutes
Cooking time: 30 minutes
Servings: 4

Ingredients:
- 1 red onion, chopped
- 1 pound turkey breast, skinless, boneless and cubed
- 2 cups broccoli florets
- 1 teaspoon cumin, ground
- 3 garlic cloves, minced
- 2 tablespoons olive oil
- 14 ounces coconut milk
- A pinch of black pepper
- ¼ cup cilantro, chopped

Directions:
1. Heat up a pot with the oil over medium heat, add the onion and the garlic, stir and sauté for 5 minutes.
2. Add the turkey, toss and brown for 5 minutes.
3. Add the broccoli and the rest of the ingredients, bring to a simmer over medium heat and cook for 20 minutes.
4. Divide the mix between plates and serve.

Nutrition: calories 438, fat 32.9, fiber 4.7, carbs 16.8, protein 23.5

Cloves Chicken

Preparation time: 10 minutes
Cooking time: 30 minutes
Servings: 4

Ingredients:
- 1 pound chicken breast, skinless, boneless and cubed
- 1 cup low-sodium chicken stock
- 1 tablespoons avocado oil
- 2 teaspoons cloves, ground
- 1 yellow onion, chopped
- 2 teaspoons sweet paprika
- 3 tomatoes, cubed
- A pinch of salt and black pepper
- ½ cup parsley, chopped

Directions:
1. Heat up a pan with the oil over medium heat, add the onion and sauté for 5 minutes.
2. Add the chicken and brown for 5 minutes more.
3. Add the stock and the rest of the ingredients, bring to a simmer and cook over medium heat for 20 minutes more.
4. Divide the mix between plates and serve.

Nutrition: calories 324, fat 12.3, fiber 5, carbs 33.10, protein 22.4

Chicken with Ginger Artichokes

Preparation time: 10 minutes
Cooking time: 30 minutes
Servings: 4

Ingredients:
- 2 chicken breasts, skinless, boneless and halved
- 1 tablespoon ginger, grated
- 1 cup canned tomatoes, no-salt-added, chopped
- 10 ounces canned artichokes, no-salt-added, drained and quartered
- 2 tablespoons lemon juice
- 2 tablespoons olive oil
- A pinch of black pepper

Directions:
1. Heat up a pan with the oil over medium heat, add the ginger and the artichokes, toss and cook for 5 minutes.
2. Add the chicken and cook for 5 minutes more.
3. Add the rest of the ingredients, bring to a simmer and cook for 20 minutes more.
4. Divide everything between plates and serve.

Nutrition: calories 300, fat 14.5, fiber 5.3, carbs 16.4, protein 15.1

Turkey and Peppercorns Mix

Preparation time: 10 minutes
Cooking time: 30 minutes
Servings: 4

Ingredients:
- ½ tablespoon black peppercorns
- 1 tablespoon olive oil
- 1 pound turkey breast, skinless, boneless and cubed
- 1 cup low-sodium chicken stock
- 3 garlic cloves, minced
- 2 tomatoes, cubed
- A pinch of black pepper
- 2 tablespoons spring onions, chopped

Directions:
1. Heat up a pan with the oil over medium heat, add the garlic and the turkey and brown for 5 minutes.
2. Add the peppercorns and the rest of the ingredients, bring to a simmer and cook over medium heat for 25 minutes.
3. Divide the mix between plates and serve.

Nutrition: calories 313, fat 13.3, fiber 7, carbs 23.4, protein 16

Chicken Thighs and Rosemary Veggies

Preparation time: 10 minutes
Cooking time: 40 minutes
Servings: 4

Ingredients:
- 2 pounds chicken breasts, skinless, boneless and cubed
- 1 carrot, cubed
- 1 celery stalk, chopped
- 1 tomato, cubed
- 2 small red onions, sliced
- 1 zucchini, cubed
- 2 garlic cloves, minced
- 1 tablespoon rosemary, chopped
- 2 tablespoons olive oil
- Black pepper to the taste
- ½ cup low-sodium veggie stock

Directions:
1. Heat up a pan with the oil over medium heat, add the onions and the garlic, stir and sauté for 5 minutes.
2. Add the chicken, toss and brown it for 5 minutes more.
3. Add the carrot and the other ingredients, toss, bring to a simmer and cook over medium heat for 30 minutes.
4. Divide the mix between plates and serve.

Nutrition: calories 325, fat 22.5, fiber 6.1, carbs 15.5, protein 33.2

Chicken with Carrots and Cabbage

Preparation time: 10 minutes
Cooking time: 25 minutes
Servings: 4

Ingredients:
- 1 pound chicken breast, skinless, boneless and cubed
- 2 tablespoons olive oil
- 2 carrots, peeled and grated
- 1 teaspoon sweet paprika
- ½ cup low-sodium veggie stock
- 1 red cabbage head, shredded
- 1 yellow onion, chopped
- Black pepper to the taste

Directions:
1. Heat up a pan with the oil over medium heat, add the onion, stir and sauté for 5 minutes.
2. Add the meat, and brown it for 5 minutes more.
3. Add the carrots and the other ingredients, toss, bring to a simmer and cook over medium heat for 15 minutes.
4. Divide everything between plates and serve.

Nutrition: calories 370, fat 22.2, fiber 5.2, carbs 44.2, protein 24.2

Eggplant and Turkey Sandwich

Preparation time: 10 minutes
Cooking time: 25 minutes
Servings: 4

Ingredients:
- 1 turkey breast, skinless, boneless and sliced into 4 pieces
- 1 eggplant, sliced into 4 slices
- Black pepper to the taste
- 1 tablespoon olive oil
- 1 tablespoon oregano, chopped
- ½ cup low sodium tomato sauce
- ½ cup low-fat cheddar cheese, shredded
- 4 whole wheat bread slices

Directions:

1. Heat up a grill over medium-high heat, add the turkey slices, drizzle half of the oil over them, sprinkle the black pepper, cook for 8 minutes on each side and transfer to a plate.
2. Arrange the eggplant slices on the heated grill, drizzle the rest of the oil over them, season with black pepper as well, cook them for 4 minutes on each side and transfer to the plate with the turkey slices as well.
3. Arrange 2 bread slices on a working surface, divide the cheese on each, divide the eggplant slices and turkey ones on each, sprinkle the oregano, drizzle the sauce all over and top with the other 2 bread slices.
4. Divide the sandwiches between plates and serve.

Nutrition: calories 280, fat 12.2, fiber 6, carbs 14, protein 12

Simple Turkey and Zucchini Tortillas

Preparation time: 10 minutes
Cooking time: 20 minutes
Servings: 4

Ingredients:
- 4 whole wheat tortillas
- ½ cup fat-free yogurt
- 1 pound turkey, breast, skinless, boneless and cut into strips
- 1 tablespoon olive oil
- 1 red onion, sliced
- 1 zucchini, cubed
- 2 tomatoes, cubed
- Black pepper to the taste

Directions:
1. Heat up a pan with the oil over medium heat, add the onion, stir and sauté for 5 minutes.
2. Add the zucchini and tomatoes, toss and cook for 2 minutes more.
3. Add the turkey meat, toss and cook for 13 minutes more.
4. Spread the yogurt on each tortilla, add divide the turkey and zucchini mix, roll, divide between plates and serve.

Nutrition: calories 290, fat 13.4, fiber 3.42, carbs 12.5, protein 6.9

Chicken with Peppers and Eggplant Pan

Preparation time: 10 minutes
Cooking time: 25 minutes
Servings: 4

Ingredients:
- 2 chicken breasts, skinless, boneless and cubed
- 1 red onion, chopped
- 2 tablespoons olive oil
- 1 eggplant, cubed
- 1 red bell pepper, cubed
- 1 yellow bell pepper, cubed
- Black pepper to the taste
- 2 cups coconut milk

Directions:
4. Heat up a pan with the oil over medium-high heat, add the onion, stir and cook for 3 minutes.
5. Add the bell peppers, toss and cook for 2 minutes more.
6. Add the chicken and the other ingredients, toss, bring to a simmer and cook over medium heat for 20 minutes more.
7. Divide everything between plates and serve.

Nutrition: calories 310, fat 14.7, fiber 4, carbs 14.5, protein 12.6

Balsamic Baked Turkey

Preparation time: 10 minutes
Cooking time: 40 minutes
Servings: 4

Ingredients:
- 1 big turkey breast, skinless, boneless and sliced
- 2 tablespoons balsamic vinegar
- 1 tablespoon olive oil
- 2 garlic cloves, minced
- 1 tablespoon Italian seasoning
- Black pepper to the taste
- 1 tablespoon cilantro, chopped

Directions:
1. In a baking dish, mix the turkey with the vinegar, the oil and the other ingredients, toss, introduce in the oven at 400 degrees F and bake for 40 minutes.
2. Divide everything between plates and serve with a side salad.

Nutrition: calories 280, fat 12.7, fiber 3, carbs 22.1, protein 14

Cheddar Turkey Mix

Preparation time: 10 minutes
Cooking time: 1 hour
Servings: 4

Ingredients:

- 1 pound turkey breast, skinless, boneless and sliced
- 2 tablespoons olive oil
- 1 cup canned tomatoes, no-salt-added, chopped
- Black pepper to the taste
- 1 cup fat-free cheddar cheese, shredded
- 2 tablespoons parsley, chopped

Directions:

1. Grease a baking dish with the oil, arrange the turkey slices into the pan, spread the tomatoes over them, season with black pepper, sprinkle the cheese and parsley on top, introduce in the oven at 400 degrees F and bake for 1 hour.
2. Divide everything between plates and serve.

Nutrition: calories 350, fat 13.1, fiber 4, carbs 32.4, protein 14.65

Parmesan Turkey

Preparation time: 10 minutes
Cooking time: 23 minutes
Servings: 4

Ingredients:
- 1 pound turkey breast, skinless, boneless and cubed
- 1 tablespoon olive oil
- ½ cup low-fat parmesan, grated
- 2 shallots, chopped
- 1 cup coconut milk
- Black pepper to the taste

Directions:
1. Heat up a pan with the oil over medium-high heat, add the shallots, toss and cook for 5 minutes.
2. Add the meat, coconut milk, and black pepper, toss and cook over medium heat for 15 minutes more.
3. Add the parmesan, cook for 2-3 minutes, divide everything between plates and serve.

Nutrition: calories 320, fat 11.4, fiber 3.5, carbs 14.3, protein 11.3

Creamy Chicken and Shrimp Mix

Preparation time: 10 minutes
Cooking time: 14 minutes
Servings: 4

Ingredients:
- 1 tablespoon olive oil
- 1 pound chicken breast, skinless, boneless and cubed
- ¼ cup low-sodium chicken stock
- 1 pound shrimp, peeled and deveined
- ½ cup coconut cream
- 1 tablespoon cilantro, chopped

Directions:
1. Heat up a pan with the oil over medium heat, add the chicken, toss and cook for 8 minutes.
2. Add the shrimp and the other ingredients, toss, cook everything for 6 minutes more, divide into bowls and serve.

Nutrition: calories 370, fat 12.3, fiber 5.2, carbs 12.6, protein 8

Basil Turkey and Hot Asparagus Mix

Preparation time: 10 minutes
Cooking time: 40 minutes
Servings: 4

Ingredients:
- 1 pound turkey breast, skinless, and cut into strips
- 1 cup coconut cream
- 1 cup low-sodium chicken stock
- 2 tablespoons parsley, chopped
- 1 bunch asparagus, trimmed and halved
- 1 teaspoon chili powder
- 2 tablespoons olive oil
- A pinch of sea salt and black pepper

Directions:
1. Heat up a pan with the oil over medium-high heat, add the turkey and some black pepper, toss and cook for 5 minutes.
2. Add the asparagus, chili powder and the other ingredients, toss, bring to a simmer and cook over medium heat for 30 minutes more.
3. Divide everything between plates and serve.

Nutrition: calories 290, fat 12.10, fiber 4.6, carbs 12.7, protein 24

Cashew Turkey Medley

Preparation time: 10 minutes
Cooking time: 40 minutes
Servings: 4

Ingredients:

- 1 pound turkey breast, skinless, boneless and cubed
- 1 cup cashews, chopped
- 1 yellow onion, chopped
- ½ tablespoon olive oil
- Black pepper to the taste
- ½ teaspoon sweet paprika
- 2 and ½ tablespoons cashew butter
- ¼ cup low-sodium chicken stock
- 1 tablespoon cilantro, chopped

Directions:

1. Heat up a pan with the oil over medium-high heat, add the onion, stir and sauté for 5 minutes.
2. Add the meat and brown it for 5 minutes more.
3. Add the rest of the ingredients, toss, bring to a simmer and cook over medium heat for 30 minutes.
4. Divide the whole mix between plates and serve.

Nutrition: calories 352, fat 12.7, fiber 6.2, carbs 33.2, protein 13.5

Turkey and Berries

Preparation time: 10 minutes
Cooking time: 35 minutes
Servings: 4

Ingredients:
- 2 pounds turkey breasts, skinless, boneless and cubed
- 1 tablespoon olive oil
- 1 red onion, chopped
- 1 cup cranberries
- 1 cup low-sodium chicken stock
- ¼ cup cilantro, chopped
- Black pepper to the taste

Directions:
1. Heat up a pot with the oil over medium-high heat, add the onion, stir and sauté for 5 minutes.
2. Add the meat, berries and the other ingredients, bring to a simmer and cook over medium heat fro 30 minutes more.
3. Divide the mix between plates and serve.

Nutrition: calories 293, fat 7.3, fiber 2.8, carbs 14.7, protein 39.3

Five Spice Chicken Breast

Preparation time: 5 minutes
Cooking time: 35 minutes
Servings: 4

Ingredients:
- 1 cup tomatoes, crushed
- 1 teaspoon five spice
- 2 chicken breast halves, skinless, boneless and halved
- 1 tablespoon avocado oil
- 2 tablespoons coconut aminos
- Black pepper to the taste
- 1 tablespoons hot pepper
- 1 tablespoon cilantro, chopped

Directions:
1. Heat up a pan with the oil over medium heat, add the meat and brown it for 2 minutes on each side.
2. Add the tomatoes, five spice and the other ingredients, bring to a simmer and cook over medium heat for 30 minutes.
3. Divide the whole mix between plates and serve.

Nutrition: calories 244, fat 8.4, fiber 1.1, carbs 4.5, protein 31

Turkey with Spiced Greens

Preparation time: 10 minutes
Cooking time: 17 minutes
Servings: 4

Ingredients:
- 1 pound turkey breast, boneless, skinless and cubed
- 1 cup mustard greens
- 1 teaspoon nutmeg, ground
- 1 teaspoon allspice, ground
- 1 yellow onion, chopped
- Black pepper to the taste
- 1 tablespoon olive oil

Directions:
1. Heat up a pan with the oil over medium-high heat, add the onion and the meat and brown for 5 minutes.
2. Add the rest of the ingredients, toss, cook over medium heat for 12 minutes more, divide between plates and serve.

Nutrition: calories 270, fat 8.4, fiber 8.32, carbs 33.3, protein 9

Chicken and Chili Mushrooms

Preparation time: 10 minutes
Cooking time: 20 minutes
Servings: 4

Ingredients:
- 2 chicken breasts, skinless, boneless and halved
- ½ pound white mushrooms, halved
- 1 tablespoon olive oil
- 1 cup canned tomatoes, no-salt-added, chopped
- 2 tablespoons almonds, chopped
- 2 tablespoons olive oil
- ½ teaspoon chili flakes
- Black pepper to the taste

Directions:
1. Heat up a pan with the oil over medium-high heat, add the mushrooms, toss and sauté for 5 minutes.
2. Add the meat, toss and cook for 5 minutes more.
3. Add the tomatoes and the other ingredients, bring to a simmer and cook over medium heat for 10 minutes.
4. Divide the mix between plates and serve.

Nutrition: calories 320, fat 12.2, fiber 5.3, carbs 33.3, protein 15

Chili Chicken and Tomatoes Artichokes

Preparation time: 10 minutes
Cooking time: 20 minutes
Servings: 4

Ingredients:
- 2 red chilies, chopped
- 1 tablespoon olive oil
- 1 yellow onion, chopped
- 1 pound chicken breasts, skinless, boneless and cubed
- 1 cup tomatoes, crushed
- 10 ounces canned artichoke hearts, drained and quartered
- Black pepper to the taste
- ½ cup low-sodium chicken stock
- 2 tablespoons lime juice

Directions:
1. Heat up a pan with the oil over medium heat, add the onion and the chilies, stir and sauté for 5 minutes.
2. Add the meat, toss and brown for 5 minutes more.
3. Add the rest of the ingredients, bring to a simmer over medium heat and cook for 10 minutes.
4. Divide the mix between plates and serve.

Nutrition: calories 280, fat 11.3, fiber 5, carbs 14.5, protein 13.5

Chicken and Beets Mix

Preparation time: 10 minutes
Cooking time: 0 minutes
Servings: 4

Ingredients:
- 1 carrot, shredded
- 2 beets, peeled and shredded
- ½ cup avocado mayonnaise
- 1 cup smoked chicken breast, skinless, boneless, cooked and shredded
- 1 teaspoon chives, chopped

Directions:
1. In a bowl, combine the chicken with the beets and the other ingredients, toss and serve right away.

Nutrition: calories 288, fat 24.6, fiber 1.4, carbs 6.5, protein 14

Turkey with Celery Salad

Preparation time: 4 minutes
Cooking time: 0 minutes
Servings: 4

Ingredients:
- 2 cups turkey breast, skinless, boneless, cooked and shredded
- 1 cup celery stalks, chopped
- 2 spring onions, chopped
- 1 cup black olives, pitted and halved
- 1 tablespoon olive oil
- 1 teaspoon lime juice
- 1 cup fat-free yogurt

Directions:
1. In a bowl, combine the turkey with the celery and the other ingredients, toss and serve cold.

Nutrition: calories 157, fat 8, fiber 2, carbs 10.8, protein 11.5

Chicken Thighs and Grapes Mix

Preparation time: 10 minutes
Cooking time: 40 minutes
Servings: 4

Ingredients:
- 1 carrot, cubed
- 1 yellow onion, sliced
- 1 tablespoon olive oil
- 1 cup tomatoes, cubed
- ¼ cup low-sodium chicken stock
- 2 garlic cloves, chopped
- 1 pound chicken thighs, skinless and boneless
- 1 cup green grapes
- Black pepper to the taste

Directions:
1. Grease a baking pan with the oil, arrange the chicken thighs inside and add the other ingredients on top.
2. Bake at 390 degrees F for 40 minutes, divide between plates and serve.

Nutrition: calories 289, fat 12.1, fiber 1.7, carbs 10.3, protein 33.9

Turkey and Lemon Barley

Preparation time: 5 minutes
Cooking time: 55 minutes
Servings: 4

Ingredients:

- 1 tablespoon olive oil
- 1 turkey breast, skinless, boneless and sliced
- Black pepper to the taste
- 2 celery stalks, chopped
- 1 red onion, chopped
- 2 cups low-sodium chicken stock
- ½ cup barley
- 1 teaspoon lemon zest, grated
- 1 tablespoon lemon juice
- 1 tablespoon chives, chopped

Directions:

1. Heat up a pot with the oil over medium-high heat, add the meat and the onion, toss and brown for 5 minutes.
2. Add the celery and the other ingredients, toss, bring to a simmer, reduce heat to medium, simmer for 50 minutes, divide into bowls and serve.

Nutrition: calories 150, fat 4.5, fiber 4.9, carbs 20.8, protein 7.5

Turkey with Beets and Radish Mix

Preparation time: 10 minutes
Cooking time: 35 minutes
Servings: 4

Ingredients:
- 1 turkey breast, skinless, boneless and cubed
- 2 red beets, peeled and cubed
- 1 cup radishes, cubed
- 1 red onion, chopped
- ¼ cup low-sodium chicken stock
- Black pepper to the taste
- 1 tablespoon olive oil
- 2 tablespoon chives, chopped

Directions:
1. Heat up a pan with the oil over medium-high heat, add the meat and the onion, toss and brown for 5 minutes.
2. Add the beets, radishes and the other ingredients, bring to a simmer and cook over medium heat for 30 minutes more.
3. Divide the mix between plates and serve.

Nutrition: calories 113, fat 4.4, fiber 2.3, carbs 10.4, protein 8.8

Garlic Pork Mix

Preparation time: 10 minutes
Cooking time: 45 minutes
Servings: 8

Ingredients:
- 2 pounds pork meat, boneless and cubed
- 1 red onion, chopped
- 1 tablespoon olive oil
- 3 garlic cloves, minced
- 1 cup low-sodium beef stock
- 2 tablespoons sweet paprika
- Black pepper to the taste
- 1 tablespoon chives, chopped

Directions:
1. Heat up a pan with the oil over medium heat, add the onion and the meat, toss and brown for 5 minutes.
2. Add the rest of the ingredients, toss, reduce heat to medium, cover and cook for 40 minutes.
3. Divide the mix between plates and serve.

Nutrition: calories 407, fat 35.4, fiber 1, carbs 5, protein 14.9

Paprika Pork with Carrots

Preparation time: 10 minutes
Cooking time: 30 minutes
Servings: 4

Ingredients:

- 1 pound pork stew meat, cubed
- ¼ cup low-sodium veggie stock
- 2 carrots, peeled and sliced
- 2 tablespoons olive oil
- 1 red onion, sliced
- 2 teaspoons sweet paprika
- Black pepper to the taste

Directions:

1. Heat up a pan with the oil over medium heat, add the onion, stir and sauté for 5 minutes.
2. Add the meat, toss and brown for 5 minutes more.
3. Add the rest of the ingredients, bring to a simmer and cook over medium heat for 20 minutes.
4. Divide the mix between plates and serve.

Nutrition: calories 328, fat 18.1, fiber 1.8, carbs 6.4, protein 34

Ginger Pork and Onions

Preparation time: 10 minutes
Cooking time: 35 minutes
Servings: 4

Ingredients:
- 2 red onions, sliced
- 2 green onions, chopped
- 1 tablespoon olive oil
- 2 teaspoons ginger, grated
- 4 pork chops
- 3 garlic cloves, chopped
- Black pepper to the taste
- 1 carrot, chopped
- 1 cup low sodium beef stock
- 2 tablespoons tomato paste
- 1 tablespoon cilantro, chopped

Directions:
1. Heat up a pan with the oil over medium heat, add the green and red onions, toss and sauté them for 3 minutes.
2. Add the garlic and the ginger, toss and cook for 2 minutes more.
3. Add the pork chops and cook them for 2 minutes on each side.
4. Add the rest of the ingredients, bring to a simmer and cook over medium heat for 25 minutes more.
5. Divide the mix between plates and serve.

Nutrition: calories 332, fat 23.6, fiber 2.3, carbs 10.1, protein 19.9

Cumin Pork

Preparation time: 10 minutes
Cooking time: 45 minutes
Servings: 4

Ingredients:
- ½ cup low-sodium beef stock
- 2 tablespoons olive oil
- 2 pounds pork stew meat, cubed
- 1 teaspoon coriander, ground
- 2 teaspoons cumin, ground
- Black pepper to the taste
- 1 cup cherry tomatoes, halved
- 4 garlic cloves, minced
- 1 tablespoon cilantro, chopped

Directions:
1. Heat up a pan with the oil over medium heat, add the garlic and the meat, toss and brown for 5 minutes.
2. Add the stock and the other ingredients, bring to a simmer and cook over medium heat for 40 minutes.
3. Divide everything between plates and serve.

Nutrition: calories 559, fat 29.3, fiber 0.7, carbs 3.2, protein 67.4

Pork and Greens Mix

Preparation time: 10 minutes
Cooking time: 20 minutes
Servings: 4

Ingredients:
- 2 tablespoons balsamic vinegar
- 1/3 cup coconut aminos
- 1 tablespoon olive oil
- 4 ounces mixed salad greens
- 1 cup cherry tomatoes, halved
- 4 ounces pork stew meat, cut into strips
- 1 tablespoon chives, chopped

Directions:
1. Heat up a pan with the oil over medium heat, add the pork, aminos and the vinegar, toss and cook for 15 minutes.
2. Add the salad greens and the other ingredients, toss, cook for 5 minutes more, divide between plates and serve.

Nutrition: calories 125, fat 6.4, fiber 0.6, carbs 6.8, protein 9.1

Thyme Pork Pan

Preparation time: 10 minutes
Cooking time: 25 minutes
Servings: 4

Ingredients:
- 1 pound pork butt, trimmed and cubed
- 1 tablespoon olive oil
- 1 yellow onion, chopped
- 3 garlic cloves, minced
- 1 tablespoon thyme, dried
- 1 cup low-sodium chicken stock
- 2 tablespoons low-sodium tomato paste
- 1 tablespoon cilantro, chopped

Directions:
1. Heat up a pan with the oil over medium-high heat, add the onion and the garlic, toss and cook for 5 minutes.
2. Add the meat, toss and cook for 5 more minutes.
3. Add the rest of the ingredients, toss, bring to a simmer, reduce heat to medium and cook the mix for 15 minutes more.
4. Divide the mix between plates and serve right away.

Nutrition: calories 281, fat 11.2, fiber 1.4, carbs 6.8, protein 37.1

Marjoram Pork and Zucchinis

Preparation time: 10 minutes
Cooking time: 30 minutes
Servings: 4

Ingredients:
- 2 pounds pork loin boneless, trimmed and cubed
- 2 tablespoons avocado oil
- ¾ cup low-sodium veggie stock
- ½ tablespoon garlic powder
- 1 tablespoon marjoram, chopped
- 2 zucchinis, roughly cubed
- 1 teaspoon sweet paprika
- Black pepper to the taste

Directions:
1. Heat up a pan with the oil over medium-high heat, add the meat, garlic powder and the marjoram, toss and cook for 10 minutes.
2. Add the zucchinis and the other ingredients, toss, bring to a simmer, reduce heat to medium and cook the mix for 20 minutes more.
3. Divide everything between plates and serve.

Nutrition: calories 359, fat 9.1, fiber 2.1, carbs 5.7, protein 61.4

Spiced Pork

Preparation time: 10 minutes
Cooking time: 8 hours
Servings: 4

Ingredients:
- 3 tablespoons olive oil
- 2 pounds pork shoulder roast
- 2 teaspoons sweet paprika
- 1 teaspoon garlic powder
- 1 teaspoon onion powder
- 1 teaspoon nutmeg, ground
- 1 teaspoon allspice, ground
- Black pepper to the taste
- 1 cup low-sodium veggie stock

Directions:
1. In your slow cooker, combine the roast with the oil and the other ingredients, toss, put the lid on and cook on Low for 8 hours.
2. Slice the roast, divide it between plates and serve with the cooking juices drizzled on top.

Nutrition: calories 689, fat 57.1, fiber 1, carbs 3.2, protein 38.8

Coconut Pork and Celery

Preparation time: 10 minutes
Cooking time: 35 minutes
Servings: 4

Ingredients:
- 2 pounds pork stew meat, cubed
- 2 tablespoons olive oil
- 1 cup low-sodium veggie stock
- 1 celery stalk, chopped
- 1 teaspoon black peppercorns
- 2 shallots, chopped
- 1 tablespoon chives, chopped
- 1 cup coconut cream
- Black pepper to the taste

Directions:
1. Heat up a pan with the oil over medium heat, add the shallots and the meat, toss and brown for 5 minutes.
2. Add the celery and the other ingredients, toss, bring to a simmer and cook over medium heat for 30 minutes more.
3. Divide everything between plates and serve right away.

Nutrition: calories 690, fat 43.3, fiber 1.8, carbs 5.7, protein 6.2

Pork and Tomatoes Mix

Preparation time: 10 minutes
Cooking time: 30 minutes
Servings: 4

Ingredients:
- 2 garlic cloves, minced
- 2 pounds pork stew meat, ground
- 2 cups cherry tomatoes, halved
- 1 tablespoon olive oil
- Black pepper to the taste
- 1 red onion, chopped
- ½ cup low-sodium veggie stock
- 2 tablespoons low-sodium tomato paste
- 1 tablespoon parsley, chopped

Directions:
1. Heat up a pan with the oil over medium heat, add the onion and the garlic, toss and sauté for 5 minutes.
2. Add the meat and brown it for 5 minutes more.
3. Add the rest of the ingredients, toss, bring to a simmer, cook over medium heat for 20 minutes more, divide into bowls and serve.

Nutrition: calories 558, fat 25.6, fiber 2.4, carbs 10.1, protein 68.7

Sage Pork Chops

Preparation time: 10 minutes
Cooking time: 35 minutes
Servings: 4

Ingredients:
- 4 pork chops
- 2 tablespoons olive oil
- 1 teaspoon smoked paprika
- 1 tablespoon sage, chopped
- 2 garlic cloves, minced
- 1 tablespoon lemon juice
- Black pepper to the taste

Directions:
1. In a baking dish, combine the pork chops with the oil and the other ingredients, toss, introduce in the oven and bake at 400 degrees F for 35 minutes.
2. Divide the pork chops between plates and serve with a side salad.

Nutrition: calories 263, fat 12.4, fiber 6, carbs 22.2, protein 16

Thai Pork and Eggplant

Preparation time: 10 minutes
Cooking time: 30 minutes
Servings: 4

Ingredients:
- 1 pound pork stew meat, cubed
- 1 eggplant, cubed
- 1 tablespoon coconut aminos
- 1 teaspoon five spice
- 2 garlic cloves, minced
- 2 Thai chilies, chopped
- 2 tablespoons olive oil
- 2 tablespoons low-sodium tomato paste
- 1 tablespoon cilantro, chopped
- ½ cup low-sodium veggie stock

Directions:
1. Heat up a pan with the oil over medium-high heat, add the garlic, chilies and the meat and brown for 6 minutes.
2. Add the eggplant and the other ingredients, bring to a simmer and cook over medium heat for 24 minutes.
3. Divide the mix between plates and serve.

Nutrition: calories 320, fat 13.4, fiber 5.2, carbs 22.8, protein 14

Pork and Lime Scallions

Preparation time: 10 minutes
Cooking time: 30 minutes
Servings: 4

Ingredients:
- 2 tablespoons lime juice
- 4 scallions, chopped
- 1 pound pork stew meat, cubed
- 2 garlic cloves, minced
- 2 tablespoons olive oil
- Black pepper to the taste
- ½ cup low-sodium veggie stock
- 1 tablespoon cilantro, chopped

Directions:
1. Heat up a pan with the oil over medium heat, add the scallions and the garlic, toss and cook for 5 minutes.
2. Add the meat, toss and cook for 5 minutes more.
3. Add the rest of the ingredients, bring to a simmer and cook over medium heat for 20 minutes.
4. Divide the mix between plates and serve.

Nutrition: calories 273, fat 22.4, fiber 5, carbs 12.5, protein 18

Balsamic Pork

Preparation time: 10 minutes
Cooking time: 30 minutes
Servings: 4

Ingredients:
- 1 red onion, sliced
- 1 pound pork stew meat, cubed
- 2 red chilies, chopped
- 2 tablespoons balsamic vinegar
- ½ cup coriander leaves, chopped
- Black pepper to the taste
- 2 tablespoons olive oil
- 1 tablespoon low-sodium tomato sauce

Directions:
1. Heat up a pan with the oil over medium heat, add the onion and the chilies, toss and cook for 5 minutes.
2. Add the meat, toss and cook for 5 minutes more.
3. Add the rest of the ingredients, toss, bring to a simmer and cook over medium heat for 20 minutes more.
4. Divide everything between plates and serve right away.

Nutrition: calories 331, fat 13.3, fiber 5, carbs 22.7, protein 17

Pesto Pork

Preparation time: 10 minutes
Cooking time: 36 minutes
Servings: 4

Ingredients:
- 2 tablespoons olive oil
- 2 spring onions, chopped
- 1 pound pork chops
- 2 tablespoons basil pesto
- 1 cup cherry tomatoes, cubed
- 2 tablespoons low-sodium tomato paste
- ½ cup parsley, chopped
- ½ cup low-sodium veggie stock
- Black pepper to the taste

Directions:
1. Heat up a pan with the olive oil over medium-high heat, add the spring onions and the pork chops, and brown for 3 minutes on each side.
2. Add the pesto and the other ingredients, toss gently, bring to a simmer and cook over medium heat for 30 minutes more.
3. Divide everything between plates and serve.

Nutrition: calories 293, fat 11.3, fiber 4.2, carbs 22.2, protein 14

Pork and Parsley Peppers

Preparation time: 10 minutes
Cooking time: 1 hour
Servings: 4

Ingredients:

- 1 green bell pepper, chopped
- 1 red bell pepper, chopped
- 1 yellow bell pepper, chopped
- 1 red onion, chopped
- 1 pound pork chops
- 1 tablespoon olive oil
- Black pepper to the taste
- 26 ounces canned tomatoes, no-salt-added and chopped
- 2 tablespoons parsley, chopped

Directions:

1. Grease a roasting pan with the oil, arrange the pork chops inside and add the other ingredients on top.
2. Bake at 390 degrees F for 1 hour, divide everything between plates and serve.

Nutrition: calories 284, fat 11.6, fiber 2.6, carbs 22.2, protein 14

Cumin Lamb Mix

Preparation time: 10 minutes
Cooking time: 25 minutes
Servings: 4

Ingredients:
- 1 tablespoon olive oil
- 1 red onion, chopped
- 1 cup cherry tomatoes, halved
- 1 pound lamb stew meat, ground
- 1 tablespoon chili powder
- Black pepper to the taste
- 2 teaspoons cumin, ground
- 1 cup low-sodium veggie stock
- 2 tablespoons cilantro, chopped

Directions:
1. Heat up the a pan with the oil over medium-high heat, add the onion, lamb and chili powder, toss and cook for 10 minutes.
2. Add the rest of the ingredients, toss, cook over medium heat for 15 minutes more.
3. Divide into bowls and serve.

Nutrition: calories 320, fat 12,7, fiber 6, carbs 14.3, protein 22

Pork with Radishes and Green Beans

Preparation time: 10 minutes
Cooking time: 35 minutes
Servings: 4

Ingredients:
- 1 pound pork stew meat, cubed
- 1 cup radishes, cubed
- ½ pound green beans, trimmed and halved
- 1 yellow onion, chopped
- 1 tablespoon olive oil
- 2 garlic cloves, minced
- 1 cup canned tomatoes, no-salt-added and chopped
- 2 teaspoons oregano, dried
- Black pepper to the taste

Directions:
1. Heat up a pan with the oil over medium-high heat, add the onion and the garlic, toss and cook for 5 minutes.
2. Add the meat, toss and cook for 5 minutes more.
3. Add the rest of the ingredients, bring to a simmer and cook over medium heat for 25 minutes.
4. Divide everything into bowls and serve.

Nutrition: calories 289, fat 12, fiber 8, carbs 13.2, protein 20

Fennel Lamb and Mushrooms

Preparation time: 10 minutes
Cooking time: 40 minutes
Servings: 4

Ingredients:
- 1 pound lamb shoulder, boneless and cubed
- 8 white mushrooms, halved
- 2 tablespoons olive oil
- 1 yellow onion, chopped
- 2 garlic cloves, minced
- 1 an ½ tablespoons fennel powder
- Black pepper to the taste
- A bunch of scallions, chopped
- 1 cup low-sodium veggie stock

Directions:
1. Heat up a pan with the oil over medium heat, add the onion and the garlic, toss and cook for 5 minutes.
2. Add the meat and the mushrooms, toss and cook for 5 minutes more.
3. Add the other ingredients, toss, bring to a simmer and cook over medium heat for 30 minutes.
4. Divide the mix into bowls and serve.

Nutrition: calories 290, fat 15.3, fiber 7, carbs 14.9, protein 14

Pork and Spinach Pan

Preparation time: 10 minutes
Cooking time: 30 minutes
Servings: 4

Ingredients:
- 1 pound pork, ground
- 2 tablespoons olive oil
- 1 red onion, chopped
- ½ pound baby spinach
- 4 garlic cloves, minced
- ½ cup low-sodium veggie stock
- ½ cup canned tomatoes, no-salt-added, chopped
- Black pepper to the taste
- 1 tablespoon chives, chopped

Directions:
1. Heat up a pan with the oil over medium-high heat, add the onion and the garlic, toss and cook for 5 minutes.
2. Add the meat, toss and brown for 5 minutes more.
3. Add the rest of the ingredients except the spinach, toss, bring to a simmer, reduce heat to medium and cook for 15 minutes.
4. Add the spinach, toss, cook the mix for another 5 minutes, divide everything into bowls and serve.

Nutrition: calories 270, fat 12, fiber 6, carbs 22.2, protein 23

Pork with Avocados

Preparation time: 10 minutes
Cooking time: 15 minutes
Servings: 4

Ingredients:
- 2 cups baby spinach
- 1 pound pork steak, cut into strips
- 1 tablespoon olive oil
- 1 cup cherry tomatoes, halved
- 2 avocados, peeled, pitted and cut into wedges
- 1 tablespoon balsamic vinegar
- ½ cup low-sodium veggie stock

Directions:
1. Heat up a pan with the oil over medium-high heat, add the meat, toss and cook for 10 minutes.
2. Add the spinach and the other ingredients, toss, cook for 5 minutes more, divide into bowls and serve.

Nutrition: calories 390, fat 12.5, fiber 4, carbs 16.8, protein 13.5

Pork and Apples Mix

Preparation time: 10 minutes
Cooking time: 40 minutes
Servings: 4

Ingredients:
- 2 pounds pork stew meat, cut into strips
- 2 green apples, cored and cut into wedges
- 2 garlic cloves, minced
- 2 shallots, chopped
- 1 tablespoon sweet paprika
- ½ teaspoon chili powder
- 2 tablespoons avocado oil
- 1 cup low-sodium chicken stock
- Black pepper to the taste
- A pinch of red chili pepper flakes

Directions:
1. Heat up a pan with the oil over medium heat, add the shallots and the garlic, toss and sauté for 5 minutes.
2. Add the meat and brown for another 5 minutes.
3. Add the apples and the other ingredients, toss, bring to a simmer and cook over medium heat for 30 minutes more.
4. Divide everything between plates and serve.

Nutrition: calories 365, fat 7, fiber 6, carbs 15.6, protein 32.4

Cinnamon Pork Chops

Preparation time: 10 minutes
Cooking time: 1 hour and 10 minutes
Servings: 4

Ingredients:
- 4 pork chops
- 2 tablespoons olive oil
- 2 garlic cloves, minced
- ¼ cup low-sodium veggie stock
- 1 tablespoon cinnamon powder
- Black pepper to the taste
- 1 teaspoon chili powder
- ½ teaspoon onion powder

Directions:
1. In a roasting pan, combine the pork chops with the oil and the other ingredients, toss, introduce in the oven and bake at 390 degrees F for 1 hour and 10 minutes.
2. Divide the pork chops between plates and serve with a side salad.

Nutrition: calories 288, fat 5.5, fiber 6, carbs 12.7, protein 23

Coconut Pork Chops

Preparation time: 10 minutes
Cooking time: 20 minutes
Servings: 4

Ingredients:
- 2 tablespoons olive oil
- 4 pork chops
- 1 yellow onion, chopped
- 1 tablespoon chili powder
- 1 cup coconut milk
- ¼ cup cilantro, chopped

Directions:
1. Heat up a pan with the oil over medium-high heat, add the onion and the chili powder, toss and sauté for 5 minutes.
2. Add the pork chops and brown them for 2 minutes on each side.
3. Add the coconut milk, toss, bring to a simmer and cook over medium heat for 11 minutes more.
4. Add the cilantro, toss, divide everything into bowls and serve.

Nutrition: calories 310, fat 8, fiber 6, carbs 16.7, protein 22.1

Pork with Peaches Mix

Preparation time: 10 minutes
Cooking time: 25 minutes
Servings: 4

Ingredients:
- 2 pounds pork tenderloin, roughly cubed
- 2 peaches, stones removed and cut into quarters
- ¼ teaspoon onion powder
- 2 tablespoons olive oil
- ¼ teaspoon smoked paprika
- ¼ cup low-sodium veggie stock
- Black pepper to the taste

Directions:
1. Heat up a pan with the oil over medium heat, add the meat, toss and cook for 10 minutes.
2. Add the peaches and the other ingredients, toss, bring to a simmer and cook over medium heat for 15 minutes more.
3. Divide the whole mix between plates and serve.

Nutrition: calories 290, fat 11.8, fiber 5.4, carbs 13.7, protein 24

Cocoa Lamb and Radishes

Preparation time: 10 minutes
Cooking time: 35 minutes
Servings: 4

Ingredients:
- ½ cup low-sodium veggie stock
- 1 pound lamb stew meat, cubed
- 1 cup radishes, cubed
- 1 tablespoon cocoa powder
- Black pepper to the taste
- 1 yellow onion, chopped
- 1 tablespoon olive oil
- 2 garlic cloves, minced
- 1 tablespoon parsley, chopped

Directions:
1. Heat up a pan with the oil over medium-high heat, add the onion and the garlic, toss and sauté for 5 minutes.
2. Add the meat, toss and brown for 2 minutes on each side.
3. Add the stock and the other ingredients, toss, bring to a simmer and cook over medium heat for 25 minutes more.
4. Divide everything between plates and serve.

Nutrition: calories 340, fat 12.4, fiber 9.3, carbs 33.14, protein 20

Lemon Pork and Artichokes

Preparation time: 10 minutes
Cooking time: 25 minutes
Servings: 4

Ingredients:
- 2 pounds pork stew meat, cut into strips
- 2 tablespoons avocado oil
- 1 tablespoon lemon juice
- 1 tablespoon lemon zest, grated
- 1 cup canned artichokes, drained and cut into quarters
- 1 red onion, chopped
- 2 garlic cloves, minced
- ½ teaspoon chili powder
- Black pepper to the taste
- 1 teaspoon sweet paprika
- 1 jalapeno, chopped
- ¼ cup low-sodium veggie stock
- ¼ cup rosemary, chopped

Directions:
1. Heat up a pan with the oil over medium-high heat, add the onion and the garlic, toss and sauté for 4 minutes.
2. Add the meat, artichokes, chili powder, the jalapeno and the paprika, toss and cook for 6 minutes more.
3. Add the rest of the ingredients, toss, bring to a simmer and cook over medium heat for 15 minutes more.
4. Divide the whole mix into bowls and serve.

Nutrition: calories 350, fat 12, fiber 4.3, carbs 35.7, protein 14.5

Pork with Cilantro Sauce

Preparation time: 10 minutes
Cooking time: 20 minutes
Servings: 4

Ingredients:
- 2 pounds pork stew meat, roughly cubed
- 1 cup cilantro leaves
- 4 tablespoons olive oil
- 1 tablespoon pine nuts
- 1 tablespoon fat-free parmesan, grated
- 1 tablespoon lemon juice
- 1 teaspoon chili powder
- Black pepper to the taste

Directions:
1. In a blender, combine the cilantro with the pine nuts, 3 tablespoons oil, parmesan and lemon juice and pulse well.
2. Heat up a pan with the remaining oil over medium heat, add the meat, chili powder and the black pepper, toss and brown for 5 minutes.
3. Add the cilantro sauce, and cook over medium heat for 15 minutes more, stirring from time to time.
4. Divide the pork between plates and serve right away.

Nutrition: calories 270, fat 6.6, fiber 7, carbs 12.6, protein 22.4

Pork with Mango Mix

Preparation time: 10 minutes
Cooking time: 25 minutes
Servings: 4

Ingredients:
- 2 shallots, chopped
- 2 tablespoons avocado oil
- 1 pound pork stew meat, cubed
- 1 mango, peeled and roughly cubed
- 2 garlic cloves, minced
- 1 cup tomatoes, and chopped
- Black pepper to the taste
- ½ cup basil, chopped

Directions:
1. Heat up a pan with the oil over medium heat, add the shallots and the garlic, toss and cook for 5 minutes.
2. Add the meat, toss and cook for 5 minutes more.
3. Add the rest of the ingredients, toss, bring to a simmer and cook over medium heat for 15 minutes more.
4. Divide the mix into bowls and serve.

Nutrition: calories 361, fat 11, fiber 5.1, carbs 16.8, protein 22

Rosemary Pork and Lemon Sweet Potatoes

Preparation time: 10 minutes
Cooking time: 35 minutes
Servings: 4

Ingredients:
- 1 red onion, cut into wedges
- 2 sweet potatoes, peeled and cut into wedges
- 4 pork chops
- 1 tablespoon rosemary, chopped
- 1 tablespoon lemon juice
- 2 teaspoons olive oil
- Black pepper to the taste
- 2 teaspoons thyme, chopped
- ½ cup low-sodium veggie stock

Directions:
1. In a roasting pan, combine the pork chops with the potatoes, onion and the other ingredients and toss gently.
2. Bake at 400 degrees F for 35 minutes, divide everything between plates and serve.

Nutrition: calories 410, fat 14.7, fiber 14.2, carbs 15.3, protein 33.4

Pork with Chickpeas

Preparation time: 10 minutes
Cooking time: 25 minutes
Servings: 4

Ingredients:
- 1 pound pork stew meat, cubed
- 1 cup canned chickpeas, no-salt-added, drained
- 1 yellow onion, chopped
- 1 tablespoon olive oil
- Black pepper to the taste
- 10 ounces canned tomatoes, no-salt-added and chopped
- 2 tablespoons cilantro, chopped

Directions:
1. Heat up a pan with the oil over medium-high heat, add the onion, toss and sauté for 5 minutes.
2. Add the meat, toss and cook for 5 minutes more.
3. Add the rest of the ingredients, toss, simmer over medium heat for 15 minutes, divide everything into bowls and serve.

Nutrition: calories 476, fat 17.6, fiber 10.2, carbs 35.7, protein 43.8

Lamb Chops with Kale

Preparation time: 10 minutes
Cooking time: 35 minutes
Servings: 4

Ingredients:
- 1 cup kale, torn
- 1 pound lamb chops
- ½ cup low-sodium veggie stock
- 2 tablespoons low-sodium tomato paste
- 1 yellow onion, sliced
- 1 tablespoon olive oil
- A pinch of black pepper

Directions:
1. Grease a roasting pan with the oil, arrange the lamb chops inside, also add the kale and the other ingredients and toss gently.
2. Bake everything at 390 degrees F for 35 minutes, divide between plates and serve.

Nutrition: calories 275, fat 11.8, fiber 1.4, carbs 7.3, protein 33.6

Chili Lamb

Preparation time: 10 minutes
Cooking time: 45 minutes
Servings: 4

Ingredients:

- 2 pounds lamb stew meat, cubed
- 1 tablespoon avocado oil
- 1 teaspoon chili powder
- 1 teaspoon hot paprika
- 2 red onions, roughly chopped
- 1 cup low-sodium veggie stock
- ½ cup low-sodium tomato sauce
- 1 tablespoon cilantro, chopped

Directions:

1. Heat up a pot with the oil over medium heat, add the onion and the meat and brown for 10 minutes.
2. Add the chili powder and the other ingredients except the cilantro, toss, bring to a simmer and cook over medium heat for 35 minutes more.
3. Divide the mix into bowls and serve with the cilantro sprinkled on top.

Nutrition: calories 463, fat 17.3, fiber 2.3, carbs 8.4, protein 65.1

Pork with Paprika Leeks

Preparation time: 10 minutes
Cooking time: 45 minutes
Servings: 4

Ingredients:
- 2 pounds pork stew meat, roughly cubed
- 2 leeks, sliced
- 2 tablespoons olive oil
- 2 garlic cloves, minced
- 1 teaspoon sweet paprika
- 1 tablespoon parsley, chopped
- 1 cup low-sodium veggie stock
- Black pepper to the taste

Directions:
1. Heat up a pan with the oil over medium heat, add the leeks, garlic and the paprika, toss and cook for 10 minutes.
2. Add the meat and brown it for 5 minutes more.
3. Add the remaining ingredients, toss, simmer over medium heat for 30 minutes, divide everything into bowls and serve.

Nutrition: calories 577, fat 29.1, fiber 1.3, carbs 8.2, protein 67.5

Pork Chops and Snow Peas

Preparation time: 10 minutes
Cooking time: 25 minutes
Servings: 4

Ingredients:
- 4 pork chops
- 2 tablespoons olive oil
- 2 shallots, chopped
- 1 cup snow peas
- 1 cup low-sodium veggie stock
- 2 tablespoons no-salt-added tomato paste
- 1 tablespoon parsley, chopped

Directions:
1. Heat up a pan with the oil over medium heat, add the shallots, toss and sauté for 5 minutes.
2. Add the pork chops and brown for 2 minutes on each side.
3. Add the rest of the ingredients, bring to a simmer and cook over medium heat for 15 minutes.
4. Divide the mix between plates and serve.

Nutrition: calories 357, fat 27, fiber 1.9, carbs 7.7, protein 20.7

Pork and Mint Corn

Preparation time: 10 minutes
Cooking time: 1 hour
Servings: 4

Ingredients:
- 4 pork chops
- 1 cup low-sodium veggie stock
- 1 cup corn
- 1 tablespoon mint, chopped
- 1 teaspoons sweet paprika
- Black pepper to the taste
- 1 tablespoon olive oil

Directions:
1. Put the pork chops in a roasting pan, add the rest of the ingredients, toss, introduce in the oven and bake at 380 degrees F for 1 hour.
2. Divide everything between plates and serve.

Nutrition: calories 356, fat 14, fiber 5.4, carbs 11.0, protein 1

Dill Lamb

Preparation time: 10 minutes
Cooking time: 25 minutes
Servings: 4

Ingredients:
- Juice of 2 limes
- 1 tablespoon lime zest, grated
- 1 tablespoon dill, chopped
- 2 garlic cloves, minced
- 2 tablespoons olive oil
- 2 pounds lamb meat, cubed
- 1 cup cilantro, chopped
- Black pepper to the taste

Directions:
1. Heat up a pan with the oil over medium-high heat, add the garlic and the meat and brown for 4 minutes on each side.
2. Add the lime juice and the other ingredients and cook for 15 minutes more stirring often.
3. Divide everything between plates and serve.

Nutrition: calories 370, fat 11.7, fiber 4.2, carbs 8.9, protein 20

Allspice Pork Chops and Olives

Preparation time: 10 minutes
Cooking time: 35 minutes
Servings: 4

Ingredients:

- 4 pork chops
- 2 tablespoons olive oil
- 1 cup kalamata olives, pitted and halved
- 1 teaspoon allspice, ground
- ¼ cup coconut milk
- 1 yellow onion, chopped
- 1 tablespoon chives, chopped

Directions:

1. Heat up a pan with the oil over medium heat, add the onion and the meat and brown for 4 minutes on each side.
2. Add the rest of the ingredients, toss gently, introduce in the oven and bake at 390 degrees F for 25 minutes more.
3. Divide everything between plates and serve.

Nutrition: calories 290, fat 10, fiber 4.4, carbs 7.8, protein 22

Italian Lamb Chops

Preparation time: 10 minutes
Cooking time: 30 minutes
Servings: 4

Ingredients:
- 4 lamb chops
- 1 tablespoon oregano, chopped
- 1 tablespoon olive oil
- 1 yellow onion, chopped
- 2 tablespoons low-fat parmesan, grated
- 1/3 cup low sodium veggie stock
- Black pepper to the taste
- 1 teaspoon Italian seasoning

Directions:
1. Heat up a pan with the oil over medium-high heat, add the lamb chops and the onion and brown for 4 minutes on each side.
2. Add the rest of the ingredients except the cheese and toss.
3. Sprinkle the cheese on top, introduce the pan in the oven and bake at 350 degrees F for 20 minutes.
4. Divide everything between plates and serve.

Nutrition: calories 280, fat 17, fiber 5.5, carbs 11.2, protein 14

Pork and Oregano Rice

Preparation time: 10 minutes
Cooking time: 35 minutes
Servings: 4

Ingredients:
- 1 tablespoon olive oil
- 1 pound pork stew meat, cubed
- 1 tablespoon oregano, chopped
- 1 cup white rice
- 2 cups low-sodium chicken stock
- Black pepper to the taste
- 2 garlic cloves, minced
- Juice of ½ lemon
- 1 tablespoon cilantro, chopped

Directions:
1. Heat up a pot with the oil over medium heat, add the meat and the garlic and brown for 5 minutes.
2. Add the rice, the stock and the other ingredients, bring to a simmer and cook over medium heat for 30 minutes.
3. Divide everything between plates and serve.

Nutrition: calories 330, fat 13, fiber 5.2, carbs 13.4, protein 22.2

Pork Meatballs

Preparation time: 10 minutes
Cooking time: 30 minutes
Servings: 4

Ingredients:
- 3 tablespoons almond flour
- 2 tablespoons avocado oil
- 2 egg, whisked
- Black pepper to the taste
- 2 pounds pork, ground
- 1 tablespoon cilantro, chopped
- 10 ounces canned tomato sauce, no-salt-added

Directions:
1. In a bowl, combine the pork with the flour and the other ingredients except the sauce and the oil, stir well and shape medium meatballs out of this mix.
2. Heat up a pan with the oil over medium heat, add the meatballs and brown for 3 minutes on each side.
   Add the sauce, toss gently, bring to a simmer and cook over medium heat for 20 minutes more.
3. Divide everything into bowls and serve.

Nutrition: calories 332, fat 18, fiber 4, carbs 14.3, protein 25

Pork and Endives

Preparation time: 10 minutes
Cooking time: 35 minutes
Servings: 4

Ingredients:

- 1 pound pork stew meat, cubed
- 2 endives, trimmed and shredded
- 1 cup low-sodium beef stock
- 1 teaspoon chili powder
- A pinch of black pepper
- 1 red onion, chopped
- 1 tablespoon olive oil

Directions:

1. Heat up a pan with the oil over medium heat, add the onion and the endives, toss and cook for 5 minutes.
2. Add the meat, toss and cook for 5 minutes more.
3. Add the rest of the ingredients, bring to a simmer and cook over medium heat for 25 minutes more.
4. Divide everything between plates and serve.

Nutrition: calories 330, fat 12.6, fiber 4.2, carbs 10, protein 22

Pork and Chives Radish

Preparation time: 10 minutes
Cooking time: 35 minutes
Servings: 4

Ingredients:
- 1 cup radishes, cubed
- 1 pound pork stew meat, cubed
- 1 tablespoon olive oil
- 1 red onion, chopped
- 1 cup canned tomatoes, no-salt-added, crushed
- 1 tablespoon chives, chopped
- 2 garlic cloves, minced
- Black pepper to the taste
- 1 teaspoon balsamic vinegar

Directions:
1. Heat up a pan with the oil over medium heat, add the onion and the garlic, stir and cook for 5 minutes.
2. Add the meat and brown for 5 minutes more.
3. Add the radishes and the other ingredients, bring to a simmer and cook over medium heat for 25 minutes more.
4. Divide everything into bowls and serve.

Nutrition: calories 274, fat 14, fiber 3.5, carbs 14.8, protein 24.1

Mint Meatballs and Spinach Sauté

Preparation time: 10 minutes
Cooking time: 25 minutes
Servings: 4

Ingredients:
- 1 pound pork stew meat, ground
- 1 yellow onion, chopped
- 1 egg, whisked
- 1 tablespoon mint, chopped
- Black pepper to the taste
- 2 garlic cloves, minced
- 2 tablespoons olive oil
- 1 cup cherry tomatoes, halved
- 1 cup baby spinach
- ½ cup low-sodium veggie stock

Directions:
1. In a bowl, combine the meat with the onion and the other ingredients except the oil, cherry tomatoes and the spinach, stir well and shape medium meatballs out of this mix.
2. Heat up a pan with the olive oil over medium-high heat, add the meatballs and cook them for 5 minutes on each side.
3. Add the spinach, tomatoes and the stock, toss, simmer everything for 15 minutes.
4. Divide everything into bowls and serve.

Nutrition: calories 320, fat 13.4, fiber 6, carbs 15.8, protein 12

Meatballs and Coconut Sauce

Preparation time: 10 minutes
Cooking time: 20 minutes
Servings: 4

Ingredients:
- 2 pounds pork, ground
- Black pepper to the taste
- ¾ cup almond flour
- 2 eggs, whisked
- 1 tablespoon parsley, chopped
- 2 red onions, chopped
- 2 tablespoons olive oil
- ½ cup coconut cream
- Black pepper to the taste

Directions:
1. In a bowl, mix the pork with the almond flour and the other ingredients except the onions, oil and the cream, stir well and shape medium meatballs out of this mix.
2. Heat up a pan with the oil over medium heat, add the onions, stir and sauté for 5 minutes.
3. Add the meatballs, and cook for 5 minutes more.
4. Add coconut cream, bring to a simmer, cook everything for 10 minutes more, divide into bowls and serve.

Nutrition: calories 435, fat 23, fiber 14, carbs 33.2, protein 12.65

Turmeric Pork and Lentils

Preparation time: 10 minutes
Cooking time: 25 minutes
Servings: 4

Ingredients:
- 1 pound pork stew meat, cubed
- ½ cup tomato sauce, no-salt-added
- 1 yellow onion, chopped
- 2 tablespoons olive oil
- 1 cup canned lentils, no-salt-added, drained
- 1 teaspoon curry powder
- 1 teaspoon turmeric powder
- Black pepper to the taste

Directions:
1. Heat up a pan with the oil over medium-high heat, add the onion and the meat and brown for 5 minutes.
2. Add the sauce and the other ingredients, toss, cook over medium heat for 20 minutes, divide everything into bowls and serve.

Nutrition: calories 367, fat 23, fiber 6.9, carbs 22.1, protein 22

Lamb Stir Fry

Preparation time: 10 minutes
Cooking time: 25 minutes
Servings: 4

Ingredients:
- 1 pound lamb meat, ground
- 1 tablespoon avocado oil
- 1 red bell pepper, cut into strips
- 1 red onion, sliced
- 2 tomatoes, cubed
- 1 carrot, cubed
- 2 fennel bulbs, sliced
- Black pepper to the taste
- 2 tablespoons balsamic vinegar
- 1 tablespoon cilantro, chopped

Directions:
1. Heat up a pan with the oil over medium-high heat, add the onion and the meat and brown for 5 minutes.
2. Add the bell pepper and the other ingredients, toss, cook over medium heat for 20 minutes more, divide into bowls and serve right away.

Nutrition: calories 367, fat 14.3, fiber 4.3, carbs 15.8, protein 16

Pork with Beets

Preparation time: 10 minutes
Cooking time: 30 minutes
Servings: 4

Ingredients:
- 1 pound pork meat, cubed
- 2 small beets, peeled and cubed
- 2 tablespoons olive oil
- 1 yellow onion, chopped
- 2 garlic cloves, minced
- Salt and black pepper to the taste
- ½ cup coconut cream.

Directions:
1. Heat up a pan with the oil over medium-high heat, add the onion and the garlic, stir and cook for 5 minutes.
2. Add the meat and brown for 5 minutes more.
3. Add the rest of the ingredients, bring to a simmer and cook over medium heat for 20 minutes.
4. Divide the mix between plates and serve.

Nutrition: calories 311, fat 14.3, fiber 4.5, carbs 15.2, protein 17

Lamb and Cabbage

Preparation time: 10 minutes
Cooking time: 35 minutes
Servings: 4

Ingredients:
- 2 tablespoons avocado oil
- 1 pound lamb stew meat, roughly cubed
- 1 green cabbage head, shredded
- 1 cup canned tomatoes, no-salt-added, chopped
- 1 yellow onion, chopped
- 1 teaspoon thyme, dried
- Black pepper to the taste
- 2 garlic cloves, minced

1. **Directions:**
2. Heat up a pan with the oil over medium-high heat, add the onion and garlic and sauté for 5 minutes.
3. Add the meat and brown for another 5 minutes.
4. Add the rest of the ingredients, toss, bring to a simmer and cook over medium heat for 25 minutes more.
5. Divide everything between plates and serve.

Nutrition: calories 325, fat 11, fiber 6.1, carbs 11.7, protein 16

Lamb with Corn and Okra

Preparation time: 10 minutes
Cooking time: 30 minutes
Servings: 4

Ingredients:
- 1 pound lamb stew meat, roughly cubed
- 1 yellow onion, chopped
- 2 garlic cloves, minced
- 2 tablespoons avocado oil
- 1 cup okra, chopped
- 1 cup corn
- 1 cup low-sodium veggie stock
- 1 tablespoon parsley, chopped

Directions:
1. Heat up a pan with the oil over medium-high heat, add the onion and the garlic, stir and sauté for 5 minutes.
2. Add the meat, toss and cook for 5 minutes more.
3. Add the rest of the ingredients, toss, bring to a simmer and cook over medium heat for 20 minutes.
4. Divide everything into bowls and serve.

Nutrition: calories 314, fat 12, fiber 4.4, carbs 13.3, protein 17

Mustard Tarragon Pork

Preparation time: 10 minutes
Cooking time: 8 hours
Servings: 4

Ingredients:
- 2 pounds pork roast, sliced
- 2 tablespoons olive oil
- Black pepper to the taste
- 1 tablespoon tarragon, chopped
- 2 shallots, chopped
- 1 cup low-sodium veggie stock
- 1 tablespoon thyme, chopped
- 1 tablespoon mustard

Directions:
1. In a slow cooker, combine the roast with the black pepper and the other ingredients, put the lid on and cook on Low for 8 hours.
2. Divide the pork roast between plates, drizzle the mustard sauce all over and serve.

Nutrition: calories 305, fat 14.5, fiber 5.4, carbs 15.7, protein 18

Pork with Sprouts and Capers

Preparation time: 10 minutes
Cooking time: 35 minutes
Servings: 4

Ingredients:
- 2 tablespoons olive oil
- 1 cup low-sodium veggie stock
- 2 tablespoons capers, drained
- 1 pound pork chops
- 1 cup bean sprouts
- 1 yellow onion, cut into wedges
- Black pepper to the taste

Directions:
1. Heat up a pan with the oil over medium-high heat, add the onion and the meat and brown for 5 minutes.
2. Add the rest of the ingredients, introduce the pan in the oven and bake at 390 degrees F for 30 minutes.
3. Divide everything between plates and serve.

Nutrition: calories 324, fat 12.5, fiber 6.5, carbs 22.2, protein 15.6

Pork with Brussels Sprouts

Preparation time: 10 minutes
Cooking time: 35 minutes
Servings: 4

Ingredients:
- 2 pounds pork stew meat, cubed
- ¼ cup low-sodium tomato sauce
- Black pepper to the taste
- ½ pound Brussels sprouts, halved
- 1 tablespoon olive oil
- 2 spring onions, chopped
- 1 tablespoon cilantro, chopped

Directions:
1. Heat up a pan with the oil over medium-high heat, add the onions and the sprouts and brown for 5 minutes.
2. Add the meat and the other ingredients, bring to a simmer and cook over medium heat for 30 minutes more.
3. Divide everything between plates and serve.

Nutrition: calories 541, fat 25.6, fiber 2.6, carbs 6.5, protein 68.7

Pork and Hot Green Beans Mix

Preparation time: 10 minutes
Cooking time: 20 minutes
Servings: 4

Ingredients:
- 1 yellow onion, chopped
- 2 pounds pork meat, cut into strips
- ½ pound green beans, trimmed and halved
- 1 red bell pepper, chopped
- Black pepper to the taste
- 1 tablespoon olive oil
- ¼ cup red hot chili pepper, chopped
- 1 cup low-sodium veggie stock

Directions:
1. Heat up a pan with the oil over medium-high heat, add the onion and sauté for 5 minutes.
2. Add the meat and brown for 5 minutes more.
3. Add the rest of the ingredients, toss, cook for 10 minutes over medium heat, divide between plates and serve.

Nutrition: calories 347, fat 24.8, fiber 3.3, carbs 18.1, protein 15.2

Lamb with Quinoa

Preparation time: 10 minutes
Cooking time: 30 minutes
Servings: 4

Ingredients:
   1 cup quinoa
   2 cups low-sodium chicken stock
   1 tablespoon olive oil
   1 cup coconut cream
   2 pounds lamb stew meat, cubed
   2 shallots, chopped
   2 garlic cloves, minced
   Black pepper to the taste
   A pinch of red pepper flakes, crushed

Directions:
   1. Heat up a pot with the oil over medium-high heat, add the shallots and the garlic, stir and sauté for 5 minutes.
   2. Add the meat and brown for 5 minutes more.
   3. Add the rest of the ingredients, stir, bring to a simmer, reduce heat to medium and cook for 20 minutes.
   4. Divide the mix bowls and serve.

Nutrition: calories 755, fat 37, fiber 4.4, carbs 32, protein 71.8

Lamb and Bok Choy Pan

Preparation time: 10 minutes
Cooking time: 30 minutes
Servings: 4

Ingredients:

- 1 cup low-sodium chicken stock
- 1 cup bok choy, torn
- 1 pound lamb stew meat, roughly cubed
- 2 tablespoons avocado oil
- 1 yellow onion, chopped
- 1 carrot, chopped
- Black pepper to the taste

Directions:

1. Heat up a pan with the oil over medium-high heat, add the onion and the carrot and sauté for 5 minutes.
2. Add the meat and brown for 5 minutes more.
3. Add the rest of the ingredients, bring to a simmer and cook over medium heat for 20 minutes.
4. Divide everything between plates and serve.

Nutrition: calories 360, fat 14.5, fiber 5, carbs 22.4, protein 16

Pork with Okra and Olives

Preparation time: 10 minutes
Cooking time: 35 minutes
Servings: 4

Ingredients:
- ½ cup low-sodium veggie stock
- 1 cup okra, trimmed
- 1 cup black olives, pitted and halved
- 2 tablespoons olive oil
- 4 pork chops
- 1 red onion, cut into wedges
- Black pepper to the taste
- ½ tablespoon red pepper flakes
- 3 tablespoons coconut aminos

Directions:
1. Grease a roasting pan with the oil and arrange the pork chops inside.
2. Add the rest of the ingredients, toss gently and bake at 390 degrees F for 35 minutes.
3. Divide everything between plates and serve.

Nutrition: calories 310, fat 14.6, fiber 6, carbs 20.4, protein 16

Pork and Capers Barley

Preparation time: 10 minutes
Cooking time: 35 minutes
Servings: 4

Ingredients:
- 1 cup barley
- 2 cups low-sodium chicken stock
- 1 pound pork stew meat, cubed
- 1 red onion, sliced
- 1 tablespoon olive oil
- Black pepper to the taste
- 1 teaspoon fenugreek powder
- 1 tablespoon chives, chopped
- 1 tablespoon capers, drained

Directions:
1. Heat up a pan with the oil over medium-high heat, add the onion and the meat and brown for 5 minutes.
2. Add the barley and the other ingredients, toss, bring to a simmer cook over medium heat for 30 minutes.
3. Divide everything into bowls and serve.

Nutrition: calories 447, fat 15.6, fiber 8.6, carbs 36.5, protein 39.8

Pork and Green Onions Mix

Preparation time: 10 minutes
Cooking time: 40 minutes
Servings: 5

Ingredients:
- 1 pound pork meat, cubed
- 1 tablespoon avocado oil
- 1 yellow onion, chopped
- 1 bunch green onion, chopped
- 4 garlic cloves, minced
- 1 cup low-sodium tomato sauce
- Black pepper to the taste

Directions:
1. Heat up a pan with the oil over medium-high heat, add the onion and green onions, stir and cook for 5 minutes.
2. Add the meat, stir and cook for 5 minutes more.
3. Add the rest of the ingredients, toss and cook over medium heat for 30 minutes more.
4. Divide everything into bowls and serve.

Nutrition: calories 206, fat 8.6, fiber 1.8, carbs 7.2, protein 23.4

Nutmeg Pork and Black Beans

Preparation time: 5 minutes
Cooking time: 40 minutes
Servings: 8

Ingredients:
- 2 tablespoons olive oil
- 1 cup canned black beans, no-salt-added, drained
- 1 yellow onion, chopped
- 1 cup canned tomatoes, no-salt-added, chopped
- 2 pounds pork stew meat, cubed
- 2 garlic cloves, minced
- Black pepper to the taste
- ½ teaspoon nutmeg, ground

Directions:
1. Heat up a pan with the oil over medium heat, add the onion and the garlic and sauté for 5 minutes.
2. Add the meat, toss and cook for 5 minutes more.
3. Add the rest of the ingredients, toss, bring to a simmer and cook over medium heat for 30 minutes.
4. Divide the mix into bowls and serve.

Nutrition: calories 365, fat 14.9, fiber 4.3, carbs 17.6, protein 38.8

Salmon and Peaches Salad

Preparation time: 10 minutes
Cooking time: 0 minutes
Servings: 4

Ingredients:
- 2 smoked salmon fillets, boneless, skinless and cubed
- 2 peaches, stones removed and cubed
- 1 teaspoon olive oil
- A pinch of black pepper
- 2 cups baby spinach
- ½ tablespoon balsamic vinegar
- 1 tablespoon lemon juice
- 1 tablespoon cilantro, chopped

Directions:
1. In a salad bowl, combine the salmon with the peaches and the other ingredients, toss and serve cold.

Nutrition: calories 133, fat 7.1, fiber 1.5, carbs 8.2, protein 1.7

Salmon and Dill Capers

Preparation time: 10 minutes
Cooking time: 15 minutes
Servings: 4

Ingredients:
- 2 tablespoons olive oil
- 4 salmon fillets, boneless
- 1 tablespoon capers, drained
- 1 tablespoon dill, chopped
- 1 shallot, chopped
- ½ cup coconut cream
- A pinch of black pepper

Directions:
1. Heat up a pan with the oil over medium-high heat, add the shallot and the capers, toss and sauté fro 4 minutes.
2. Add the salmon and cook it for 3 minutes on each side.
3. Add the rest of the ingredients, cook everything for 5 minutes more, divide between plates and serve.

Nutrition: calories 369, fat 25.2, fiber 0.9, carbs 2.7, protein 35.5

Salmon and Cucumber Salad

Preparation time: 10 minutes
Cooking time: 0 minutes
Servings: 4

Ingredients:
- 2 tablespoons olive oil
- ½ teaspoon lemon juice
- ½ teaspoon lemon zest, grated
- A pinch of black pepper
- 1 cup black olives, pitted and halved
- 1 cup cucumber, cubed
- ½ pound smoked salmon, boneless and cubed
- 1 tablespoon chives, chopped

Directions:
1. In a salad bowl, combine the salmon with the olives and the other ingredients, toss and serve.

Nutrition: calories 170, fat 13.1, fiber 1.3, carbs 3.2, protein 10.9

Tuna and Shallots

Preparation time: 10 minutes
Cooking time: 15 minutes
Servings: 4

Ingredients:
- 4 tuna fillets, boneless and skinless
- 1 tablespoon olive oil
- 2 shallots, chopped
- 2 tablespoons lime juice
- A pinch of black pepper
- 1 teaspoon sweet paprika
- ½ cup low-sodium chicken stock

Directions:
1. Heat up a pan with the oil over medium-high heat, add shallots and sauté for 3 minutes.
2. Add the fish and cook it for 4 minutes on each side.
3. Add the rest of the ingredients, cook everything for 3 minutes more, divide between plates and serve.

Nutrition: calories 404, fat 34.6, fiber 0.3, carbs 3, protein 21.4

Minty Cod Mix

Preparation time: 10 minutes
Cooking time: 17 minutes
Servings: 4

Ingredients:
- 2 tablespoons olive oil
- 1 tablespoon lemon juice
- 1 tablespoon mint, chopped
- 4 cod fillets, boneless
- 1 teaspoons lemon zest, grated
- A pinch of black pepper
- ¼ cup shallot, chopped
- ½ cup low-sodium chicken stock

Directions:
1. Heat up a pan with the oil over medium heat, add the shallots, stir and sauté for 5 minutes.
2. Add the cod, the lemon juice and the other ingredients, bring to a simmer and cook over medium heat for 12 minutes.
3. Divide everything between plates and serve.

Nutrition: calories 160, fat 8.1, fiber 0.2, carbs 2, protein 20.5

Cod and Tomatoes

Preparation time: 10 minutes
Cooking time: 16 minutes
Servings: 4

Ingredients:
- 2 tablespoons olive oil
- 2 garlic cloves, minced
- ½ cup low-sodium veggie stock
- 4 cod fillets, boneless
- 1 cup cherry tomatoes, halved
- 2 tablespoons lime juice
- A pinch of black pepper
- 1 tablespoon chives, chopped

Directions:
1. Heat up a pan with the oil over medium-high heat, add the garlic and the fish and cook for 3 minutes on each side.
2. Add the rest of the ingredients, bring to a simmer and cook over medium heat for 10 minutes more.
3. Divide everything between plates and serve.

Nutrition: calories 169, fat 8.1, fiber 0.8, carbs 4.7, protein 20.7

Paprika Tuna

Preparation time: 4 minutes
Cooking time: 10 minutes
Servings: 4

Ingredients:
- 2 tablespoons olive oil
- 4 tuna steaks, boneless
- 2 teaspoons sweet paprika
- ½ teaspoon chili powder
- A pinch of black pepper

Directions:
1. Heat up a pan with the oil over medium-high heat, add the tuna steaks, season with paprika, black pepper and chili powder, cook for 5 minutes on each side, divide between plates and serve with a side salad.

Nutrition: calories 455, fat 20.6, fiber 0.5, carbs 0.8, protein 63.8

Orange Cod

Preparation time: 5 minutes
Cooking time: 12 minutes
Servings: 4

Ingredients:
- 1 tablespoon parsley, chopped
- 4 cod fillets, boneless
- 1 cup orange juice
- 2 spring onions, chopped
- 1 teaspoon orange zest, grated
- 1 tablespoon olive oil
- 1 teaspoon balsamic vinegar
- A pinch of black pepper

Directions:
1. Heat up a pan with the oil over medium heat, add the spring onions, and sauté for 2 minutes.
2. Add the fish and the other ingredients, cook for 5 minutes on each side, divide everything between plates and serve.

Nutrition: calories 152, fat 4.7, fiber 0.4, carbs 7.2, protein 20.6

Basil Salmon

Preparation time: 5 minutes
Cooking time: 14 minutes
Servings: 4

Ingredients:

- 2 tablespoons olive oil
- 4 salmon fillets, skinless
- 2 garlic cloves, minced
- A pinch of black pepper
- 2 tablespoons balsamic vinegar
- 2 tablespoons basil, chopped

Directions:

1. Heat up a pan with the olive oil, add the fish and cook for 4 minutes on each side.
2. Add the rest of the ingredients, cook everything for 6 minutes more.
3. Divide everything between plates and serve.

Nutrition: calories 300, fat 18, fiber 0.1, carbs 0.6, protein 34.7

Cod and White Sauce

Preparation time: 10 minutes
Cooking time: 15 minutes
Servings: 4

Ingredients:
- 2 tablespoons olive oil
- 4 cod fillets, boneless and skinless
- 1 shallot, chopped
- ½ cup coconut cream
- 3 tablespoons non-fat yogurt
- 2 tablespoons dill, chopped
- A pinch of black pepper
- 1 garlic clove minced

Directions:
1. Heat up a pan with the oil over medium heat, add the shallots and sauté for 5 minutes.
2. Add the fish and the other ingredients, and cook for 10 minutes more.
3. Divide everything between plates and serve.

Nutrition: calories 252, fat 15.2, fiber 0.9, carbs 7.7, protein 22.3

Halibut and Radishes Mix

Preparation time: 10 minutes
Cooking time: 15 minutes
Servings: 4

Ingredients:
- 2 shallots, chopped
- 4 halibut fillets, boneless
- 1 cup radishes, halved
- 1 cup tomatoes, cubed
- 1 tablespoon olive oil
- 1 tablespoon cilantro, chopped
- 2 teaspoons lemon juice
- A pinch of black pepper

Directions:
1. Grease a roasting pan with the oil and arrange the fish inside.
2. Add the rest of the ingredients, introduce in the oven and bake at 400 degrees F for 15 minutes.
3. Divide everything between plates and serve.

Nutrition: calories 231, fat 7.8, fiber 6, carbs 11.9, protein 21.1

Almond Salmon Mix

Preparation time: 10 minutes
Cooking time: 15 minutes
Servings: 4

Ingredients:
- 2 tablespoons olive oil
- ½ cup almonds, chopped
- 4 salmon fillets, boneless
- 1 shallot, chopped
- ½ cup low-sodium veggie stock
- 2 tablespoons parsley, chopped
- Black pepper to the taste

=

Directions:
1. Heat up a pan with the oil over medium heat, add the shallot and sauté for 4 minutes.
2. Add the salmon and the other ingredients, cook for 5 minutes on each side, divide everything between plates and serve.

Nutrition: calories 240, fat 6.4, fiber 2.6, carbs 11.4, protein 15

Cod and Broccoli

Preparation time: 10 minutes
Cooking time: 20 minutes
Servings: 4

Ingredients:
- 2 tablespoons coconut aminos
- 1 pound broccoli florets
- 4 cod fillets, boneless
- 1 red onion, chopped
- 2 tablespoons olive oil
- ¼ cup low-sodium chicken stock
- Black pepper to the taste

Directions:
1. Heat up a pan with the oil over medium heat, add the onion and the broccoli and cook for 5 minutes.
2. Add the fish and the other ingredients, cook for 20 minutes more, divide everything between plates and serve.

Nutrition: calories 220, fat 14.3, fiber 6.3, carbs 16.2, protein 9

Ginger Sea Bass Mix

Preparation time: 10 minutes
Cooking time: 15 minutes
Servings: 4

Ingredients:
- 1 tablespoon balsamic vinegar
- 1 tablespoon ginger, grated
- 2 tablespoons olive oil
- Black pepper to the taste
- 4 sea bass fillets, boneless
- 1 tablespoon cilantro, chopped

Directions:
1. Heat up a pan with the oil over medium heat, add the fish and cook for 5 minutes on each side.
2. Add the rest of the ingredients, cook everything for 5 minutes more, divide everything between plates and serve.

Nutrition: calories 267, fat 11.2, fiber 5.2, carbs 14.3, protein 14.3

Salmon and Green Beans

Preparation time: 10 minutes
Cooking time: 20 minutes
Servings: 4

Ingredients:
- 2 tablespoons olive oil
- 1 cup low-sodium chicken stock
- 4 salmon fillets, boneless
- 2 garlic cloves, minced
- 1 tablespoon ginger, grated
- ½ pound green beans, trimmed and halved
- 2 teaspoons balsamic vinegar
- ¼ cup scallions, chopped

Directions:
1. Heat up a pan with the oil over medium heat, add the scallion and the garlic and sauté for 5 minutes.
2. Add the salmon and cook it for 5 minutes on each side.
3. Add the rest of the ingredients, cook everything for 5 minutes more, divide between plates and serve.

Nutrition: calories 220, fat 11.6, fiber 2, carbs 17.2, protein 9.3